Record Keeping
for Nurses and Midwives
AN ESSENTIAL GUIDE

Amanda Andrews
Bernie St Aubyn

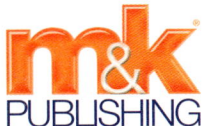

For the full range of M&K Publishing books please visit our website:
www.mkupdate.co.uk

About the authors

Amanda Andrews and Bernie St Aubyn are Senior Lecturers at Birmingham City University, where they work hard to embed record keeping into every course they teach.

They have been on a record keeping campaign for several years and this resource is the culmination of their years of clinical experience and teaching.

Record Keeping for Nurses and Midwives: An essential guide
Amanda Andrews & Bernie St Aubyn
ISBN: 978-1-905539-25-3

First published 2020

All rights reserved. No part of this publication may be reproduced, stored in a retrieval system, or transmitted in any form or by any means, electronic, mechanical, photocopying, recording or otherwise, without either the prior permission of the publishers or a licence permitting restricted copying in the United Kingdom issued by the Copyright Licensing Agency, 90 Tottenham Court Road, London, W1T 4LP. Permissions may be sought directly from M&K Publishing, phone: 01768 773030, fax: 01768 781099 or email: publishing@mkupdate.co.uk

Any person who does any unauthorised act in relation to this publication may be liable to criminal prosecution and civil claims for damages.

British Library Catalogue in Publication Data

A catalogue record for this book is available from the British Library

Notice
Clinical practice and medical knowledge constantly evolve. Standard safety precautions must be followed, but, as knowledge is broadened by research, changes in practice, treatment and drug therapy may become necessary or appropriate. Readers must check the most current product information provided by the manufacturer of each drug to be administered and verify the dosages and correct administration, as well as contraindications. It is the responsibility of the practitioner, utilising the experience and knowledge of the patient, to determine dosages and the best treatment for each individual patient. Any brands mentioned in this book are as examples only and are not endorsed by the Publisher. Neither the publisher nor the authors assume any liability for any injury and/or damage to persons or property arising from this publication.

Disclaimer
M&K Publishing cannot accept responsibility for the contents of any linked website or online resource. The existence of a link does not imply any endorsement or recommendation of the organisation or the information or views which may be expressed in any linked website or online resource. We cannot guarantee that these links will operate consistently and we have no control over the availability of linked pages.

The Publisher
To contact M&K Publishing write to:
M&K Update Ltd, The Old Bakery, St. John's Street, Keswick, Cumbria CA12 5AS
Tel: 01768 773030 | publishing@mkupdate.co.uk | www.mkupdate.co.uk

Designed and typeset by Jeremy Fisher at www.processcreative.co.uk
Printed in Scotland by Bell & Bain, Glasgow

Contents

		Page
	Preface	vii
Chapter **1**	Introduction to record keeping principles	1
Chapter **2**	Court-proofing your documents	7
Chapter **3**	Record keeping in practice	11
Chapter **4**	Electronic patient record systems	15
Chapter **5**	Test your record keeping knowledge	17
	Answer guide for quiz in Chapter 5	20
	References	23

Preface

For too long, record keeping has been considered an 'add-on' to nursing care. Often regarded as less important than the care itself, it may only be given a nominal amount of time at the end of a shift. Yet the Nursing and Midwifery Council's *Code* (2018) clearly states that record keeping is a professional obligation and an *integral* part of nursing care. Furthermore, Standard 10 within the professional standard 'Practice effectively' includes six key statements on the keeping of clear and accurate records related to practice. This guide takes a three-pronged approach to record keeping, looking at the clinical aspects, the professional obligations and the legal requirements.

We begin by introducing the general principles of record keeping and the legal implications which make it imperative that records are well documented and court-proof (in other words, accepted by the legal profession). As nurses caring for patients, we need to adhere to the law; and correctly documented records can be used as legal evidence to prove what care was given, and when and how it was given. For over a decade, we have trained undergraduate nurses on the principles of record keeping and encouraged students to reflect and think critically and professionally about their records. Previous students, who are now qualified, have told us that they still remember a live simulation session during their training. They recall the image of Barrister Bernie, the guardian angel of record keeping, sitting on their shoulder, reminding them that 'if it's not written down, it's not done'!

We have campaigned for improved record keeping in the nursing profession for many years – and there are many myths and half-truths about record keeping that we hope this guide will help to demolish. It will replace the need for an 'angel on your shoulder'. Keep it close and use it well, as it will keep you *safe*.

Amanda Andrews and **Bernie St Aubyn,** 2020

Chapter 1
Introduction to record keeping principles

The records we keep are an important communication tool, providing continuity of care between different healthcare professionals. They demonstrate whether or not a nurse is using evidence-based practice and they also provide evidence that can be used in court about the care a nurse has delivered. So there is a fundamental need for nurses to keep records.

Regardless of whether the information is handwritten or inputted electronically, you need to consider both *how* you are writing and *what* you are writing. Remember 'if it's not written down, it wasn't done'.

This section will introduce you to the key principles of record keeping, which can be applied across all healthcare fields and used with any paperwork or electronic template.

Record keeping and the four stages of the nursing process

Each of the four stages of the nursing process has specific documentation associated with it.
Firstly, the patient is assessed and information is recorded and various risk assessments are completed.

Secondly, a care plan relevant to the individual patient's problems is written or printed. This outlines the care to be given by all the nursing staff to mitigate the problems that have been identified for the patient (as the nursing process involves taking a problem-solving approach).

Thirdly, the care is carried out and various charts are used to record and monitor the patient's progress.

Finally, the care that has been delivered is evaluated and this evaluation is recorded on an evaluation sheet or discharge summary.

The need for good-quality records

We have established that there is a need for records and that the quality of your records has an impact on the quality of your clinical practice. Good-quality records promote high standards of clinical care by facilitating:

- Continuity of care
- Good communication and dissemination of information between members of the multidisciplinary team (MDT)
- An accurate account of treatment, care planning and delivery of care
- The ability to detect problems at an early stage
- The ability to respond to complaints or legal processes.

Good-quality records should include:

- A full account of the patient's assessment and the care you have planned and provided
- Relevant information about the condition of the patient at any given time and the measures you have taken to respond to their needs
- Evidence that you have understood and honoured your duty of care
- Evidence that you have taken all *reasonable* steps to care for the patient; and no action or omission on your part has compromised their safety
- A record of arrangements you have made for the patient's continuing care.

Underlying record keeping principles

Now we'll consider the underlying principles of record keeping that can be applied to all clinical areas of practice. No matter where you work, or what type of records your organisation keeps, applying these principles will keep your patients safe and keep *you* safe.

Records need to be:
- Legible
- Signed (print name and job title alongside signature)
- Dated and timed
- Accurate and clear
- Factual, avoiding:
  - Unnecessary abbreviations
  - Jargon
  - Meaningless phrases
  - Offensive statements
  - Irrelevant speculation.

Legible and signed

You need to *own* your records and you do this by signing them. However, not everyone's signature is recognisable or legible so best practice dictates that you also *print* your name alongside your signature. In order to identify yourself professionally, some organisations will also ask you to write your designation and your NMC PIN number or work identification number.

Dated and timed

The correct way to write the date in the UK incorporates both letters and numbers. The rule is two numbers for the date, the first three letters of the month and the year in full (e.g. '21 Feb 2020' or '05 May 2018'. This avoids any risk of confusing the date and the month, which occurs if all numbers are used.

When writing times, the 24-hour clock reduces the confusion between AM and PM – so *use it.*

Accurate and clear

You should have confidence in your own records. Never make things up, as this is fraudulent. Simply document things that you have done. Clarity is increased by writing things in full. It only takes a few more seconds to do this and could be potentially lifesaving. Any entry will be made more helpful by including numbers and names, alongside the date and times.

Unnecessary abbreviations and jargon

Jargon refers to words and phrases that only a specific set of people understand, often those in a particular profession. Using jargon clearly hinders communication. In nursing practice, we need to ensure that our notes help (rather than hinder) communication with others. So, as well as being accurate and clear, make sure you write your records for *all* your potential readers. Ask yourself if they could all understand what you have written?

We also need to consider the use of abbreviations. Certain professional abbreviations (like NHS and GP) are commonly recognised. However, any terms that are not widely known should be avoided. If their use is unavoidable, they should be accompanied by a glossary of terms to aid understanding and therefore communication.

Meaningless phrases

Time is a valuable commodity so let's not waste it by writing meaningless phrases in our documents. Let's try to make every entry count. Sometimes notes are full of vague phrases such as 'has had a settled day' or 'patient appears well'. These phrases give no specific detail about a patient's condition at any given time and therefore do not add anything to the clinical picture of the patient's condition.

Offensive statements

Beware of using offensive statements in your records, as these can damage the therapeutic relationship. There is always a more neutral and straightforward way to record information. Always remember who might be reading your notes and write for all possible readers. For instance, how would you feel if you read your own notes and found yourself being described as 'obese' or 'very overweight'? Many people would take offence at such a statement. It is far better (and more neutral) to calculate the person's Body Mass Index (BMI) and write it down as a number. The information is still being given but the value judgement has now been removed from this potentially upsetting issue.

Irrelevant speculation

Do not jump to conclusions or add your own thoughts and opinions about a situation. Good records only record the facts. For example, if you write an entry that says the patient threw themselves out of bed because they were looking for attention, the only factual element is that the patient fell out of bed. You have no insight into their mind-set and cannot state with any certainty what their state of mind was when this happened.

Other key record keeping principles

Every entry you make in your records should also be:

- Contemporaneous – written as soon as possible after an event has occurred, providing current information on the care and condition of the patient
- Written clearly, in such a manner that the text cannot be erased
- Written so that any alterations or additions are dated, timed and signed, in such a way that the original entry can still be clearly read
- Written, wherever possible, with the involvement of the patient or carer and in terms that the patient can understand
- Readable on photocopies – made using black, oil-based ink.

Most common problems found in nursing documents

The NMC has identified these as the most common problems that occur when completing nursing documents – and it's worth reflecting on them in relation to your own record keeping practices:

- Absence of clarity, e.g. using vague phrases like 'had a good day' or 'slept well' where the meaning is not clear
- Failure to record action taken when a problem is identified, e.g. 'is suffering increasing pain', but no record of what action was taken
- Missing information, e.g. administration of a drug not documented
- Spelling mistakes, e.g. errors in names of medications or diseases, resulting in wrong diagnosis
- Inaccurate records, e.g. changing a dressing or giving medication when the patient has not in fact received the recorded treatment (this error led to a nurse being removed from the NMC Register)
- Failure to document the care given – for instance, even if the patient's condition remains stable over time and the care does not differ (e.g. a patient in long-term residential care) an entry still needs to be made on each occasion, to record the care given
- Failure to document special needs, e.g. not recording the fact that a patient is deaf in her left ear
- Failures in communication between healthcare professionals, e.g. not documenting conversations and verbal instructions
- Too much jargon
- Failure in patient identification, e.g. not ensuring that patient information is entered on an identity band, and not transferring patient details on to clinical documents and continuation sheets
- Unprofessional terminology
- Mixing opinion with facts.

Chapter 2
Court-proofing your documents

Now let's consider your records from a legal perspective – a very different culture from that of nursing. Poor records often reflect poor practice (De Groot, Triemstra & Paans *et al.* 2018); and poor documentation often features in legal proceedings focusing on professional accountability and patient complaints, to the detriment of the nurse in the witness box.

Following good record keeping protocols will ensure that you can provide 'court-proof' professional records, written in a clear and logical fashion and acceptable to the legal profession. Court-proof records also promote good communication between healthcare professionals, demonstrate that evidence-based practice has been used, and provide robust evidence to defend the care given, should that care be disputed in a court, an NMC hearing or as part of a complaint process.

How are nursing records used in a legal context?

The legal system works in a chronological and ordered way. Your legal representative on the case will draw up a timeline of events to establish who, what, when, why, where and how the incident occurred. In order to be in the best position to defend your practice, it makes sense to keep your records complete and up-to-date so that you can provide the information required. If you remember to include **Numbers, Names, Dates and Times,** and adhere to the principles in Chapter 1, you will always be able to defend your care, as you will be able to provide clear, factual information to populate an accurate timeline. Your records will also provide the facts needed for a witness statement, should the case go to court.

Often the first sign of a potential misconduct issue is that a nurse receives a notification from the NMC. If this happens to you, you will undoubtedly be in a state of shock and fear at first. Saying 'sorry' will always help but 'actions speak louder than words'. The Nurses Defence Service UK (NDS) (2018) highly recommend that you seek legal advice as early as possible. Another course of action would be to reflect on the allegation of misconduct in line with your professional *Code*. However, the NDS UK (2018) advise that a written reflection is often not enough. In this case, you will have to collate supporting evidence, depending on the level of alleged misconduct. Your professional *Code* is an essential reference when collecting your evidence.

Professional standards and record keeping

Record keeping is integrated into all four professional standards in *The Code* (NMC 2018):
1. Prioritise people
2. Practise effectively
3. Preserve safety
4. Promote professionalism and trust.

And this clearly indicates the ongoing importance of good record keeping. However, it also provides the legal profession with ammunition to identify where our practice falls short of *The Code* (2018). Although record keeping is often seen as an unwanted chore to be performed at the end of a shift, if we are to adhere to the four standards of *The Code,* we all have to improve the quality of our record keeping.

We will now look at these four standards to identify where and how record keeping has been adopted.

Prioritise people

NMC Code 4 Act in the best interest of people at all times

- **Make sure that you get properly informed consent** *and* **document it before carrying out any action**

It is imperative not only to gain informed consent but also to document that this consent has been obtained before any care is carried out. Consent can be implied by an action. For example, if a person rolls up their sleeve for an injection, this is implied consent and their action can be recorded. It doesn't matter whether the consent is implied, verbal or written, as all forms of consent are held to be legally valid. What matters is that there is documented evidence showing that the consent has been gained.

> *If consent is highlighted as an issue – it would be essential to include this section in a written reflection on professional values.*

Practise effectively

NMC Code 7 Communicate clearly

- 7.5 Be able to communicate clearly and effectively in English

Practising effectively means ensuring the care we provide is based on the best evidence available and that this is reflected in the documents we complete.

Nurses' verbal communication is generally good and most of us consider the different languages and/or communication requirements of our patients in a culturally sensitive manner. The standard of 'practising effectively' requires us to be able to communicate clearly and effectively in English and this requires a good standard of grammar and spelling, as well as an understanding of the difference between fact and opinion.

NMC Code 8 Work cooperatively

- 8.3 Keep colleagues informed when you are sharing the care of individuals with other healthcare professionals

Records can also be an important communication tool, especially in the current climate of multi-professional working. Keeping our colleagues informed of patients' care helps to preserve everyone's safety and improves risk management.

These points could be included in any report on further training undertaken to improve communication skills and/or written skills.

Preserve patient and public safety

NMC Code 14 Be open and candid with all service users about all aspects of care and treatment, including when any mistakes or harm have taken place

- 14.3 Document all these events formally and take further action (escalate) if appropriate so they can be dealt with quickly

This standard highlights the need to preserve patient and public safety, working within the limits of our competence.

We also need to be mindful of the 'duty of candour' that obliges nurses to raise concerns immediately whenever a situation puts a patient or member of the public at risk. The professional duty of candour requires us to be open and honest about the care we deliver, to preserve safety.

Nurses are human and sometimes mistakes happen, but *The Code* explicitly states that all situations of actual or potential harm need to be formally documented as part of the process of escalating the problem so that the appropriate action can be taken. This is particularly pertinent if you believe a patient is vulnerable and needs protection.

> *Once again, these are supportive sections in relation to re-training – for example, mandatory training requirements, medication management training and perhaps safeguarding updates/courses.*

Promote professionalism and trust

NMC Code 20 Uphold the reputation of your profession at all times

- 20.1 Keep to and uphold the standards and value set out in *The Code*

The final standard of *The Code* urges us to uphold the reputation of the nursing profession. Nurses who produce high-quality documentation demonstrate a personal commitment to the standards of practice and behaviour set out in *The Code,* thereby upholding the reputation of the profession.

> *This final point could be supported by character statements from colleagues and peers as to your overall professional credibility.*

Chapter 3
Record keeping in practice

Remembering the importance of numbers, names dates and times

Having considered the general principles and the legal aspects of record keeping, we need to look at practical record keeping in the clinical setting. We cannot provide you with a 'one size fits all' method of writing your records, as each clinical setting has its own documentation requirements, and patient care is individual and person-centred. What we *can* do is give you some ideas based on clinical experience, in line with the key principles.

Legible and signed, dated and timed

As we said earlier, you need to *own* your records. A clear record of the care you have delivered needs to be identifiable as yours and provide evidence of the patient's journey. The records need to be written as soon as possible after the event and/or in line with organisational procedures.

Remember: The date is written as DD/MMM/YYYY and time is recorded using the 24-hour clock.

> 03/Mar/20XX 09:30 Mrs Smith was assisted with personal care this morning at 08:00. She requested a shower and was supported with this by myself and Health Care Assistant Sharon Powell.
>
> *A Johnson* Amanda Johnson. Staff Nurse. Ward 12

Accurate, clear and factual records

We can only report the facts and they need to be documented accurately and clearly, to reduce the risk of ambiguity. In order to develop these skills, consider using as few words as possible and only use words if you feel confident about their meaning and spelling. Also remember to avoid unnecessary abbreviations, jargon and irrelevant speculation. Always ask yourself if you can understand what you have written – and remember to 'write for the reader'!

> 03/Mar/20XX 09:30 Mrs Smith was assisted with personal care this morning at 08:00. She requested a shower and was supported with this by myself and Health Care Assistant Sharon Powell. Today, Mrs Smith has developed a red area on her left heel. It measures 1cm width (around her heel) x 1.5cm height (rising up her heel).
>
> *A Johnson* Amanda Johnson. Staff Nurse. Ward 12

Person-centred practice

Whenever possible, patients should be included in the documented entries relating to their care. What could be better than quoting what they said, in their own words? Alternatively, you can make use of numerical scales. For instance, you can report their level of pain, using a scale from 1 to 5.

> 03/Mar/20XX 09:30 Mrs Smith was assisted with personal care this morning at 08:00. She requested a shower and was supported with this by myself and Health Care Assistant Sharon Powell. Mrs Smith has today developed a red area on her left heel. It measures 1cm width (around her heel) x 1.5cm height (rising up her heel). Mrs Smith reported on a pain scale of 0 (no pain) to 5 (most severe pain) that the pain from her heel was a score of 2.
>
> *A Johnson* Amanda Johnson. Staff Nurse. Ward 12

What if I make a mistake in the patient's record?

From time to time everyone will make a documentation error, whether it's a spelling error or recording incorrect information. Remember, the key to correction is not to *hide* your mistakes. Best practice is to strike through the error and *own* it. A tip is to make the strike-through appear like a gate with a clear start and finish. This is to ensure your mistake is not extended or amended out of context. If the error is over a larger area, strike it through with a single Z-shaped annotation, starting at the first word, with the diagonal across all the text and the end point being the last word.

> 03/Mar/20XX 09:30 Mrs Smith was assisted with personal care this morning at 08:00. She requested a shower and was supported with this by myself and Health Care Assistant Sharon Powell. /Mrs Smith has today developed a red area on her right heel/ (written in error 03/Mar/20XX *A Johnson* Amanda Johnson). Mrs Smith has today developed a red area on her left heel. It measures 1cm width (around her heel) x 1.5cm height (rising up her heel). Mrs Smith reported on a pain scale of 0 (no pain) to 5 (most severe pain) that the pain from her heel was a score of 2.
>
>   *A Johnson* Amanda Johnson. Staff Nurse. Ward 12

I have recorded the issue – should I write anything else?

The Code tells us that we should always also document the actions taken to respond to the problems identified.

> 03/Mar/20XX 09:30 Mrs Smith was assisted with personal care this morning at 08:00. She requested a shower and was supported with this by myself and Health Care Assistant Sharon Powell. /Mrs Smith has today developed a red area on her right heel/ (written in error 03/Mar/20XX *A Johnson* Amanda Johnson). Mrs Smith has today developed a red area on her left heel. It measures 1cm width (around her heel) x 1.5cm height (rising up her heel). Mrs Smith reported on a pain scale of 0 (no pain) to 5 (most severe pain) that the pain from her heel was a score of 2. A protective foot pressure relieving boot was applied to Mrs Smith's left heel. 2 x 500mg Paracetamol (as per prescription chart) given to Mrs Smith at 13:00. The effectiveness of these interventions to be reviewed in 2 hours. Care plan written for new identified pressure area risk (see care plan 2).
>
>   *A Johnson* Amanda Johnson. Staff Nurse. Ward 12

I always wash my hands so do I need to bother writing that anywhere in my documentation?

One of the main issues at NMC conduct committees relates to nurses' inability to show proof of what they have done. **Remember: 'If it isn't written down – it wasn't done!'** It is the common tasks nurses do every day that they forget to record. It does not have to be recorded every time but should appear *at least once* in one of the patient's documents. If it relates to a nursing care task, the best place would be in the care plan, as an intervention.

> **Care plan interventions – those tasks we forget to record (remember to personalise it – change 'patient' to preferred given name)**
>
> 1. Introduce yourself and ask the patient what their preferred name is
> 2. Give clear instructions to the patient and gain consent to continue with the care plan
> 3. Wash hands according to local Trust policy
> 4. Maintain the patient's privacy and dignity by (add specific points here relating to clinical setting, e.g. draw curtains around patient's bed space)

We hope this chapter has given you a clear idea of how to develop your own style of record keeping.

Remember:
- **Practice makes Perfect in Practice**
- **Numbers, Names, Dates and Times**
- **'If it isn't written down – it wasn't done!'**

Chapter 4
Electronic patient record systems

Many organisations now use electronic patient record systems (EPRS). As this use steadily increases, it is essential that nurses pay more attention to the quality of their documentation (Jefferies, Johnson & Griffiths 2010). In this chapter we will consider the advantages and disadvantages of EPRS and consider how the principles described in Chapter 1 apply to this mode of record keeping.

The advantages of EPRS

Electronic patient record systems not only enable up-to-date information to be documented in a structured way, but they also allow easy access to that information. This offers the healthcare professional an instant overview of the patient's current care needs. Many EPRS save valuable time by having drop-down menus which provide standard statements that can be inserted. Meissner and Schnepp (2014) also suggest that electronic records enable care decisions to be made more quickly and easily. Firstly, an EPRS automatically stores the 'log-in data' so there is no problem identifying the originator of the records or when the record was made. However, this raises the need for passwords and SMART cards to remain private and exclusive to the person to whom they are issued (RCN 2012).

Good record keeping principles teach us to use unambiguous language to ensure that only factual, clear and accurate information is recorded and shared. EPRS help to facilitate this by using unambiguous structured language, but this only works when the system uses a recognised classification, e.g. North American Nursing Diagnosis Association (NANDA), which is tailored to specific nursing settings.

EPRS need to be accessible to all members of the multidisciplinary team to avoid any problems when nurses hand over information to other healthcare professionals. (Without good-quality record keeping, handovers can be challenging and continuity of care may be impeded.) EPRS systems are also useful for benchmarking and quality audit purposes, as the information they contain is readily accessible for re-use (De Groot, Triemstra & Paans *et al.* 2018).

The challenges of EPRS

There are some ongoing maintenance costs associated with EPRS, including staff training and updates as required. In addition, equipment needs to be purchased, updated, maintained and integrated across existing systems.

There are also operational challenges with EPRS, as these systems can make it easier for nurses *not* to think about nursing care processes. This could lead to the full description of the patient's health not being captured, as well as reduced person-centred care and a reduction in nurses' critical thinking skills. For EPRS to work well, these systems need to be developed in consultation with nursing staff. This will help ensure that various evidence-based instruments are included, covering all aspects of the nursing process.

Chapter 5
Test your record keeping knowledge

1 Identify below the reasons why we keep records
(Note: There may be more than one correct answer):

   a) As a communication tool
   b) As legal evidence
   c) Because employers tell us to
   d) Because it promotes best practice
   e) All of the above

2 Match each type of record with the correct stage of the nursing process:

Records	Nursing process
a) Admission Paperwork	a) Assessment
b) Progress Notes	b) Implementation
c) Fluid Balance Chart	c) Evaluation
d) Care Plan	d) Planning

3 Good records promote _____ care. This is an essential part of nursing practice. Choose one of the answers below to fill the blank.

| continuity of | nursing | health promotion of |

4 Where would you look for guidance on good record keeping?

   a) NMC website
   b) Health Education England website
   c) Your own Trust website

5 To meet legal requirements, does care have to be:

   a) Reasonable?
   b) Regulated?
   c) Regularly reviewed?

6 How do you demonstrate accountability for your records?

a) Date and sign them
b) Print them
c) Check them with a colleague.
d) Store them correctly

7 Where are your nursing records used as evidence?
(Note: There may be more than one correct answer):

a) A Trust Annual General Meeting
b) An NMC hearing
c) A performance review
d) A clinical supervision meeting
e) A court of law

8 Which is the most important P to protect with good records?

a) Patients
b) Practitioners
c) PIN numbers

9 Replace the *italic* words using simpler terms from the boxes below:

The patient is *tachycardic, secondary to a lower respiratory tract infection.*

short of breath	due to	double pneumonia
experiencing pain	primarily	urinary infection
has a raised pulse	and has	chest infection

10 What are the four things lawyers *love*? Complete the list below.

a) Numbers
b) ……………..
c) Dates
d) ……………..

Answers are available on p. 20.

Answer guide for quiz in Chapter 5

1. Match each type of record with the correct stage of the nursing process:

   Answers:
   As a communication tool
   As legal evidence
   Because it promotes best practice

2. Match each type of record with the correct stage of the nursing process:
   Answers:

Records	Nursing process
Admission Paperwork	Assessment
Progress Notes	Evaluation
Fluid Balance Chart	Implementation
Care Plan	Planning

3. Good records promote _____ care. This is an essential part of nursing practice. Choose one answer from the box to fill the blank.

   Answer: Good records promote **continuity of** care. This is an essential part of nursing practice.

4. Where would you look for guidance on good record keeping?

   Answer: NMC website

5. To meet legal requirements, does care have to be:

   Answer: Reasonable

6. How do you demonstrate accountability for your records?

   Answer: Date and sign them

7. Where are your nursing records used as evidence?
   (Note: There may be more than one correct answer):

   Answer:
   An NMC hearing
   A court of law

8   Which is the most important P to protect with good records?

    Answer: Patients

9   Replace the *italic* words using simpler terms from the box below:

    Answer: The patient has **a raised pulse, due to** a **chest infection.**

10 What are the four things lawyers *love*? Complete the list below.

    Answers:
    a) Numbers
    b) Names
    c) Dates
    d) Times

References

De Groot, K., Triemstra, M., Paans, W. & Francke, A. (2018). Quality criteria, instruments, and requirements for nursing documentation: A systematic review of systematic reviews. *Journal of Advanced Nursing.* **75**, 1379–93.

Jefferies, D., Johnson, M. & Griffiths, R. (2010). A meta-study of the essentials of quality nursing documentation. *International Journal of Nursing Practice.* **16**, 112–24.

Meissner, A. & Schnepp, W. (2014). Staff experiences within the implantation of computer-based nursing records in residential aged care facilities: A systematic review and synthesis of qualitative research. *BMC Medical Informatics and Decision Making.* **144**, 54.

Nurses Defence Service UK (2018). Nurses and Reflective Writing in NMC Cases (Showing Insight). https://nursesdefenceservice.com/nurses-and-reflective-writing-in-nmc-cases/ (last accessed on 10.7.2020).

Nursing and Midwifery Council (NMC) (2018). *The Code.* https://www.nmc.org.uk/standards/code/read-the-code-online/ (last accessed on 10.7.2020).

Royal College of Nursing (RCN) (2012). *Delegating Record Keeping and Countersigning Records. Guidance for Nursing Staff.* London: RCN Publications.